Peptide Guide

A Beginner's 3-Week Plan for Women to Support Hormones, Fat Loss, Skin Health, and Longevity

copyright © 2025 Isadora Kwon

All rights reserved No part of this book may be reproduced, or stored in a retrieval system, or transmitted in any form or by any means, electronic, mechanical, photocopying, recording, or otherwise, without express written permission of the publisher.

Disclaimer

By reading this disclaimer, you are accepting the terms of the disclaimer in full. If you disagree with this disclaimer, please do not read the guide.

All of the content within this guide is provided for informational and educational purposes only, and should not be accepted as independent medical or other professional advice. The author is not a doctor, physician, nurse, mental health provider, or registered nutritionist/dietician. Therefore, using and reading this guide does not establish any form of a physician-patient relationship.

Always consult with a physician or another qualified health provider with any issues or questions you might have regarding any sort of medical condition. Do not ever disregard any qualified professional medical advice or delay seeking that advice because of anything you have read in this guide. The information in this guide is not intended to be any sort of medical advice and should not be used in lieu of any medical advice by a licensed and qualified medical professional.

The information in this guide has been compiled from a variety of known sources. However, the author cannot attest to or guarantee the accuracy of each source and thus should not be held liable for any errors or omissions.

You acknowledge that the publisher of this guide will not be held liable for any loss or damage of any kind incurred as a result of this guide or the reliance on any information provided within this guide. You acknowledge and agree that you assume all risk and responsibility for any action you undertake in response to the information in this guide.

Using this guide does not guarantee any particular result (e.g., weight loss or a cure). By reading this guide, you acknowledge that there are no guarantees to any specific outcome or results you can expect.

All product names, diet plans, or names used in this guide are for identification purposes only and are the property of their respective owners. The use of these names does not imply endorsement. All other trademarks cited herein are the property of their respective owners.

Where applicable, this guide is not intended to be a substitute for the original work of this diet plan and is, at most, a supplement to the original work for this diet plan and never a direct substitute. This guide is a personal expression of the facts of that diet plan.

Where applicable, persons shown in the cover images are stock photography models and the publisher has obtained the rights to use the images through license agreements with third-party stock image companies.

Table of Contents

Introduction   7
Unlocking the Power of Peptides for Women's Health   9
    What Are Peptides and Why They Matter for Women's Health 9
    How Peptides Can Help with Hormones, Fat Loss, Skin, and Aging   10
Peptides & Women's Hormones – Balancing Estrogen, Progesterone & More   13
    Understanding Hormonal Imbalances: PCOS, Menopause, and Thyroid Issues   13
    Peptides that Regulate Hormones (e.g., BPC-157, CJC-1295, Ipamorelin)   14
    How Peptides Can Help with PMS, Perimenopause & Menopause   15
Peptides for Fat Loss & Metabolism – Boosting Energy & Burning Stubborn Fat   18
    Why Women's Metabolism Changes with Age and Hormones 18
    Peptides for Fat Loss: MOTS-c, Tesamorelin, and AOD-9604 22
    How to Stack Peptides for Fat Loss & Maintain Lean Muscle 25
Peptides for Skin Health & Anti-Aging – Collagen, Wrinkles & Hair Growth   27
    How Peptides Boost Collagen & Skin Repair   27
    Best Peptides for Anti-Aging: GHK-Cu, Thymosin Beta-4, and Epitalon   28
    Using Peptides for Hair Growth & Stronger Nails   30
Peptides for Longevity, Energy & Mood – Staying Vibrant at Any Age   34
    How Peptides Enhance Cellular Regeneration & Energy Levels 34
    Brain-Boosting Peptides for Focus, Memory & Mood   35

Peptides for Sleep & Stress Relief to Combat Burnout 39

How to Safely Get Started – Sourcing, Dosage & Legal Considerations **44**

Understanding Peptide Regulations & Safe Sourcing for Women 44

How to Dose Peptides for Maximum Benefits with Minimal Risk 46

When to Cycle Peptides & How to Monitor Your Progress 47

The 3-Week Peptide Protocol for Women's Wellness **54**

Week 1: Detailed Plan – Hormonal Reset & Energy Boost 54

Week 2 Detailed Plan – Skin Rejuvenation & Fat Loss Acceleration 59

Week 3 Detailed Plan – Longevity & Anti-Aging Optimization 63

Troubleshooting & Adjusting for Your Unique Body **69**

Recognizing Common Side Effects 69

When to Adjust Dosages 71

What to Do If You Don't See Results – Common Pitfalls & Fixes 74

Long-Term Strategies: How to Maintain Benefits & Cycle Peptides Safely 77

Conclusion **81**

FAQs **83**

References and Helpful Links **86**

Introduction

Peptides are making waves as a breakthrough in women's health, offering targeted solutions to some of the most challenging aspects of aging and wellness. These tiny amino acid chains, often referred to as the body's messengers, are harnessing the power of science to make real, visible changes from the inside out. Whether it's balancing hormones, revitalizing skin, aiding fat loss, or promoting graceful aging, peptides are proving to be a game-changer in how women approach health and beauty.

What sets peptides apart is their ability to personalize wellness. Unlike one-size-fits-all approaches, peptides work with the body's unique needs, supporting hormone regulation, collagen production, and fat-burning processes at the cellular level.

For women facing the ups and downs of hormonal imbalances, stubborn weight gain, or early signs of aging, their impact can be remarkable. Experience increased energy, healthier skin, and shedding stubborn pounds—not through quick fixes, but by supporting your body to work as it's designed to.

In this guide, we will talk about the following:

- What Are Peptides & Why They Matter for Women's Health
- Understanding Hormonal Imbalances: PCOS, Menopause, and Thyroid Issues
- Peptides for Skin Health & Anti-Aging – Collagen, Wrinkles & Hair Growth
- Peptides for Longevity, Energy & Mood – Staying Vibrant at Any Age
- How to Safely Get Started – Sourcing, Dosage & Legal Considerations
- 3-Week Peptide Protocol for Women's Wellness
- Troubleshooting & Adjusting for Your Unique Body
- Managing Side Effects & When to Adjust Dosages
- Long-Term Strategies: How to Maintain Benefits & Cycle Peptides Safely

For those ready to explore a smarter, more science-backed approach to wellness, this guide is the perfect starting point. Peptides are opening up possibilities that go beyond traditional options, offering hope, solutions, and inspiration to women who want to feel and look their best, no matter their age.

Unlocking the Power of Peptides for Women's Health

What Are Peptides and Why They Matter for Women's Health

Peptides are short chains of amino acids, the building blocks of proteins, that play a crucial role in various biological processes within the body. Think of them as messengers. These tiny molecules send important signals to cells, triggering specific actions that help maintain health and wellness. While peptides occur naturally in the body, science has discovered ways to harness and optimize them for targeted health benefits.

For women, peptides hold significant promise in addressing unique health challenges. From regulating hormone levels to improving skin health, peptides work at a cellular level to support the body in dynamic and meaningful ways.

They're not a one-size-fits-all solution but rather a tailored approach designed to meet individual needs. This makes peptides an exciting area of focus for women looking to enhance their well-being, address aging concerns, and maintain vitality as they age.

How Peptides Can Help with Hormones, Fat Loss, Skin, and Aging

Peptides shine in their ability to target specific aspects of women's health. Their versatility lies in how they interact with the body's systems, particularly in four key areas:

1. **Hormone Balance**

   Fluctuating hormones can create a domino effect, disrupting mood, sleep, energy levels, and more. Some peptides, like those that influence the production of human growth hormone (HGH), help regulate these imbalances.

   By doing so, they promote steadier energy, improved metabolism, and emotional stability. For women dealing with menopause or hormonal shifts, peptides may offer a way to bring balance back to what may feel chaotic.

2. **Fat Loss**

   Peptides play a role in boosting metabolism and breaking down fat more efficiently. For example, certain peptides stimulate the release of HGH, which is linked to improved fat-burning and lean muscle growth.

Others may help regulate appetite or increase the body's ability to use stored fat as an energy source. Women seeking healthy, sustainable weight management can find peptides to be a helpful tool in their health toolkit.

3. **Skin Health**

Healthy, glowing skin is often high on the priority list, and peptides can be a game changer in this area. These molecules support collagen production, which keeps skin firm and smooth. They also aid in repairing tissue and maintaining hydration, reducing the appearance of wrinkles and fine lines. For women wanting to slow down visible signs of aging or improve their skin's texture, peptides can offer noticeable results.

4. **Aging Gracefully**

Aging is part of life, but peptides can help make the process gentler on the body. Beyond just skin-level benefits, they support cellular repair, improve sleep quality, and enhance energy and recovery. This leads to a more youthful feeling from the inside out. Women who prioritize their long-term health will find that peptides can be a powerful ally in staying active, vibrant, and resilient through the years.

Peptides are not magic pills, but they represent what science has to offer in personalized, targeted health solutions. For women looking to take control of their health and aging process, peptides open doors to possibilities that simply weren't available before. This chapter sets the stage for understanding their incredible potential. With the right approach, peptides can be a pivotal part of optimizing health and living life to the fullest.

Peptides & Women's Hormones – Balancing Estrogen, Progesterone & More

Women's hormones are complex and often misunderstood, but they play a crucial role in overall health and well-being. Peptides offer a unique approach to hormone balance, supporting the body's natural processes and optimizing hormone levels for optimal health.

Understanding Hormonal Imbalances: PCOS, Menopause, and Thyroid Issues

Hormones work like the body's internal messengers, keeping things running smoothly. But when they get out of balance, it can feel like everything goes off track. For women, hormonal imbalances often show up as common health issues like PCOS (polycystic ovary syndrome), thyroid problems, or the roller coaster of menopause.

PCOS is a condition where women produce higher levels of certain hormones, leading to irregular periods, acne, weight struggles, and even infertility. Thyroid imbalances can make you feel either super sluggish (hypothyroidism) or overly wired (hyperthyroidism), and both can impact weight, energy, and mood.

Then there's menopause, which naturally occurs as women age but often comes with hot flashes, night sweats, mood swings, and sleep trouble due to shifting levels of estrogen and progesterone.

Hormonal imbalances like these can feel overwhelming, but there are ways to support the body in regaining balance—and peptides are one of the promising tools.

Peptides that Regulate Hormones (e.g., BPC-157, CJC-1295, Ipamorelin)

Peptides can work like targeted assistants, interacting with the body in ways that encourage hormone regulation. There's no one-size-fits-all solution, but certain peptides stand out for their ability to help balance hormones:

- *BPC-157*: BPC-157 is often used for its healing properties. It helps repair tissues and reduce inflammation, which can be hugely beneficial when hormonal imbalances are causing stress and physical discomfort. For women with gut issues or inflammatory conditions tied to hormones, BPC-157 offers strong support.

- *CJC-1295*: This peptide works by stimulating the production of human growth hormone (HGH), which can have a ripple effect throughout the body. It helps with improving metabolism, aiding fat loss, boosting energy, and supporting better sleep—all of which are crucial when hormones are out of whack.
- *Ipamorelin*: Ipamorelin also promotes the release of HGH but with fewer potential side effects. It's often used to improve recovery and energy levels. For women experiencing dips in vitality as their hormones shift, this peptide can act like a much-needed reset.

When used under the guidance of a healthcare professional, these peptides can make a meaningful difference in helping the body recover and rebalance.

How Peptides Can Help with PMS, Perimenopause & Menopause

The ups and downs of PMS, perimenopause, and menopause can impact everything from mood to quality of life. Peptides bring relief by addressing some of the underlying issues:

During PMS

For women dealing with painful cramps, mood swings, fatigue, or bloating during PMS, peptides like BPC-157 offer a promising solution. This peptide works by reducing inflammation and promoting tissue repair, which can help alleviate the discomfort caused by hormonal fluctuations.

By supporting the body's natural healing processes, BPC-157 not only helps minimize physical symptoms like cramps and bloating but may also contribute to improved mood and overall well-being. This makes it a potential game-changer for those seeking relief from the recurring challenges of PMS.

During Perimenopause

This is the transitional phase before menopause, typically occurring in a woman's 40s or early 50s, and it is marked by fluctuating hormone levels that can cause various physical and emotional changes.

Women often experience symptoms like fatigue, weight gain, mood swings, and difficulty sleeping. Peptides that regulate Human Growth Hormone (HGH), such as CJC-1295 and Ipamorelin, can provide support during this time by helping to maintain consistent energy levels, improve the body's ability to manage weight, enhance muscle tone, and promote better sleep—addressing one of the most common struggles women face during this phase of life.

During Menopause

Menopause introduces unique challenges as estrogen and progesterone levels decrease significantly, affecting various aspects of health. While peptides cannot replace these lost hormones, they can play a supportive role in maintaining overall health and resilience during this transition. For instance, peptides that stimulate collagen production may help address skin changes like dryness, thinning, or loss of elasticity, which are common during menopause.

Additionally, certain peptides can support energy levels, improve muscle tone, and even contribute to better mood regulation, helping to combat fatigue, muscle loss, and emotional fluctuations often experienced at this stage of life. By targeting specific areas, peptides can provide a holistic approach to managing menopausal symptoms and enhancing quality of life.

Peptides work on a cellular level to support balance and healing, making them an exciting option in managing hormonal shifts. They're not a cure-all, but they represent an effective, science-backed option for women wanting better control over their health.

Hormonal imbalances don't have to take over your life. With peptides as part of a broader wellness plan, it's possible to find balance and feel like yourself again. Chapter 1 lays the foundation for understanding how peptides and hormones work together to create a healthier, more harmonious body.

Peptides for Fat Loss & Metabolism – Boosting Energy & Burning Stubborn Fat

Now that we've explored the role of peptides in hormonal balance, let's dive into another common issue that people struggle with: fat loss and metabolism. Our bodies are complex systems, and many factors can impact our ability to maintain a healthy weight and energy level. Peptides offer a unique approach to supporting fat loss and boosting metabolism by working on a cellular level to optimize bodily functions.

Why Women's Metabolism Changes with Age and Hormones

Metabolism is the body's engine, converting the food you eat into the energy you need to survive and thrive. It powers virtually every function in your body, from keeping your heart beating to fueling your brain.

But as women age, many notice that maintaining a healthy weight or shedding excess fat becomes more difficult. Why does this happen? The answer lies in the intricate interplay between shifting hormones, muscle loss, and lifestyle factors.

Hormonal Changes and Their Impact

Hormones are key players in regulating metabolism and how your body stores or burns fat. For women, this balance starts to shift significantly in their 30s and continues as they age. Levels of estrogen, progesterone, and even testosterone naturally decline as part of the aging process. These hormonal changes directly affect the body's fat distribution and energy use.

- *Estrogen* plays a central role in metabolism. When levels drop, as they do with age, it can lead to an increase in fat storage, particularly around the abdominal area. This type of fat, often referred to as "visceral fat," is more stubborn and harder to lose.
- *Progesterone*, which works in harmony with estrogen, also decreases, contributing to hormonal imbalances that can impact appetite regulation and water retention.
- *Testosterone*, although present in smaller amounts in women compared to men, is vital for maintaining muscle mass. Declining testosterone levels mean muscle tissue dwindles over time, and since muscle burns more calories than fat, this reduction slows the metabolism further.

The Role of Muscle Mass

Muscles play a crucial role in keeping your metabolism humming. It's metabolically active, meaning it burns calories even when you're at rest. However, as women age, they naturally lose muscle mass (a process known as sarcopenia). This decline starts subtly in your 30s but accelerates in your 40s and beyond, significantly impacting calorie burn.

When muscle mass decreases, so does the body's overall energy requirement. This means you need fewer calories to maintain your weight, making it easier to gain weight if your eating habits don't adjust. Even consistent exercise may feel less effective as muscle strength and mass wane.

Stress, Sleep, and Cortisol

Modern life often piles on additional challenges. Stress and lack of quality sleep are two major factors that disrupt metabolism and hormones further.

High levels of stress increase **cortisol**, the stress hormone. While cortisol plays an important role in managing your body's response to stress, chronically elevated levels can encourage fat storage, particularly around the belly. At the same time, high cortisol can interfere with other hormones, like those that regulate hunger and satiety, making it harder to resist cravings or manage portions.

Sleep deprivation is another factor that worsens the problem. Poor sleep affects hormones like **ghrelin** and **leptin**, which help control hunger. When these are out of balance, you're more likely to overeat or reach for calorie-dense comfort foods. Combine that with the slowed metabolism from hormonal shifts, and the challenges of weight management intensify substantially.

All these changes, from hormonal fluctuations to muscle loss and lifestyle pressures, don't happen in isolation. They converge, making it harder for women to maintain or lose weight as they age. This doesn't just affect physical appearance; it also impacts overall health. Abdominal fat, for example, raises the risk of developing conditions like diabetes, heart disease, and other metabolic disorders.

But the story doesn't end on a bleak note. While these challenges are real, there are solutions to help your body adapt and thrive.

Supporting Your Metabolism

One promising avenue for reigniting your metabolism and improving fat-burning potential is through peptides. Peptides are short chains of amino acids that play a role in signaling and regulating various functions in the body. Some specific peptides are designed to stimulate metabolism by encouraging the breakdown of fat and helping to preserve lean muscle.

When combined with a balanced lifestyle that includes muscle-strengthening exercises, stress management techniques, and adequate sleep, peptides can complement your body's efforts to stay healthy and fit. They work with your body's natural processes, addressing some of the root causes of a slowing metabolism rather than just treating the symptoms.

Aging brings natural changes to the body, including shifts in hormone levels, muscle mass, and metabolism speed. While these adjustments can make weight management trickier for women, understanding the reasons behind these changes and taking proactive steps can make a significant difference.

By investing in approaches like resistance training, prioritizing rest, and exploring innovative solutions like peptides, you can give your metabolism the boost it needs to help you take control of your health and well-being.

Getting older doesn't mean you lose control over your body. With the right knowledge and tools, you can work with these changes—not against them—to stay strong, vibrant, and ready for life at every stage.

Peptides for Fat Loss: MOTS-c, Tesamorelin, and AOD-9604

Peptides offer targeted support by mimicking natural processes in the body to improve fat metabolism, enhance energy, and promote lean body mass. Each peptide offers unique mechanisms and benefits tailored to different fat-loss goals.

1. **MOTS-c**

   MOTS-c is a mitochondrial peptide that directly improves metabolic efficiency and energy production.

   - *How It Works*: MOTS-c targets the mitochondria, the powerhouse of the cell, boosting their ability to convert nutrients into energy. It also improves insulin sensitivity, helping the body better regulate blood sugar and avoid storing excess fat.
   - *Benefits for Women*: This peptide supports weight loss by encouraging fat-burning for energy, especially during exercise. Women experiencing hormonal-driven metabolic shifts can find MOTS-c particularly beneficial due to its insulin-regulating properties.

2. **Tesamorelin**

   Tesamorelin is a growth hormone-releasing peptide specifically known for targeting visceral fat (fat around the organs).

   - *How It Works*: Tesamorelin stimulates the natural release of growth hormone, which plays a crucial role in regulating body composition, reducing belly fat, and improving muscle tone.

- ***Benefits for Women***: By reducing visceral fat, Tesamorelin not only aids fat loss but also improves metabolic health and reduces the risk of diseases like diabetes and heart disease. Women struggling with midsection fat can benefit from its targeted effects.

3. **AOD-9604**

    Known as the "fat-burning peptide," AOD-9604 is a fragment of the growth hormone molecule selectively designed to target fat metabolism.

    - ***How It Works***: AOD-9604 enhances lipolysis (fat breakdown) and inhibits lipogenesis (formation of new fat). The result is increased fat-burning capacity without affecting hunger hormones like ghrelin.
    - ***Benefits for Women***: AOD-9604 helps women shed stubborn fat in problem areas, particularly when combined with a healthy diet and exercise routine. Its localized fat-loss effects make it appealing for body contouring purposes.

Using one or more of these peptides can significantly enhance fat metabolism and overall energy, making the weight-loss process more efficient and sustainable.

How to Stack Peptides for Fat Loss & Maintain Lean Muscle

Stacking peptides simply means using two or more peptides together to enhance their benefits. For fat loss and metabolism, strategic peptide stacking can amplify results while ensuring you maintain lean muscle.

For example, **pairing MOTS-c** with **Tesamorelin** can give you a one-two punch for fat loss. MOTS-c improves how your body uses energy, while Tesamorelin boosts HGH levels, helping with fat burning and muscle preservation. Adding **AOD-9604** to the mix can further target stubborn fat deposits while supporting a balanced metabolism.

Maintaining lean muscle is a key part of any fat-loss plan. Muscles don't just make you look toned; they also help keep your metabolism strong. To support muscle during fat loss, it's important to focus on strength training and adequate protein intake while letting peptides like Tesamorelin do their job in stimulating muscle growth and recovery.

When stacking peptides, it's crucial to follow a healthcare professional's guidance. They can recommend the right combinations, doses, and timing to suit your individual needs and goals.

Fat loss and metabolism can become trickier to manage with age, but peptides offer a smart, science-based way to turn things around. By addressing the root causes of a sluggish metabolism—like hormonal shifts and muscle loss—peptides like MOTS-c, Tesamorelin, and AOD-9604 can help women burn stubborn fat and feel energized again. When combined thoughtfully, these peptides make it possible to gain better control over your weight and rediscover a sense of vitality.

Peptides for Skin Health & Anti-Aging – Collagen, Wrinkles & Hair Growth

In this chapter, we'll delve into the role that peptides play in promoting healthy skin and anti-aging effects. Peptides have long been used in skincare products for their ability to stimulate collagen production and improve skin elasticity, resulting in reduced wrinkles and a more youthful appearance.

How Peptides Boost Collagen & Skin Repair

Collagen is the building block of youthful, elastic, and firm skin. Unfortunately, as you age, your body's natural production of collagen declines. This leads to sagging skin, wrinkles, and dryness. Peptides step in to stimulate collagen synthesis and repair skin from the inside out.

- *What Peptides Do*: Certain peptides communicate with the skin cells, encouraging them to produce more collagen and elastin. These proteins are vital for keeping your skin firm and reducing visible lines.

Peptides also aid skin repair by calming inflammation and speeding up the healing of damaged tissues.

- *Why It Helps Aging Skin*: Stimulating collagen production helps replenish what's lost over time. This can smooth wrinkles, firm sagging areas, and improve the skin's ability to retain moisture.

Key Benefits for Skin Health:

- Improved skin elasticity and resilience
- Reduced appearance of fine lines and wrinkles
- Faster wound healing and reduced redness

By incorporating peptides into your skincare routine or via targeted therapies, you can rejuvenate your skin and restore its natural glow over time.

Best Peptides for Anti-Aging: GHK-Cu, Thymosin Beta-4, and Epitalon

Not all peptides are created equal. Some stand out for their powerful anti-aging effects. Here are three of the best:

1. **GHK-Cu**

    GHK-Cu is a copper peptide widely celebrated in skincare and anti-aging science. It promotes **collagen production, improves skin elasticity, and speeds up wound healing**. This peptide also has antioxidant properties, meaning it protects your skin from damage caused by free radicals (the villains behind aging). With regular use, GHK-Cu can reduce wrinkles, smooth fine lines, and even brighten skin tone for a more youthful glow.

2. **Thymosin Beta-4**

Thymosin Beta-4 focuses on repair and regeneration. It **reduces inflammation, enhances recovery, and helps promote the growth of new blood vessels**, which improves circulation to the skin. This can lead to healthier, rejuvenated skin that appears less tired and more vibrant. This peptide is especially helpful for those with stressed or damaged skin.

3. **Epitalon**

Epitalon is known for its ability to slow down the aging process. It helps **lengthen telomeres**, which are **protective caps on the ends of your DNA**. Shortened telomeres are linked to aging, so maintaining their length can help your cells function more effectively for longer. While its anti-aging effects extend beyond just skin, users often notice firmer, smoother skin after regular use of Epitalon.

These peptides work individually and synergistically to target the signs of aging from multiple angles. Whether your goal is to reverse wrinkles, achieve a firmer complexion, or repair damaged skin, these peptides are powerful allies.

Using Peptides for Hair Growth & Stronger Nails

When you think about beauty and self-care, glowing skin might take center stage, but healthy hair and strong nails are equally important. Enter peptides, the multitasking champions that can revolutionize your haircare and nail care routines. These tiny chains of amino acids don't just work wonders on your skin; they also offer big benefits for your hair and nails.

How Peptides Promote Hair Growth

Hair growth starts from the scalp. To wake up those tired hair follicles and encourage thicker, healthier strands, peptides can be a game-changer. The key lies in their ability to deliver nutrients directly to the scalp and stimulate cellular communication.

Peptides like **copper peptides** are particularly effective in enhancing hair health. Copper peptides work by boosting blood flow to the scalp, which improves oxygen and nutrient delivery to your hair follicles. This increased circulation revitalizes dormant follicles and strengthens active ones, encouraging hair growth. Not only that, they reduce inflammation in the scalp, creating the perfect environment for hair to thrive.

Another powerful peptide often used for hair growth is acetyl tetrapeptide-3. This peptide targets the root of the problem by improving follicle anchoring and strengthening the connective tissue around the follicle base. The result? Less hair shedding and healthier, fuller locks over time.

Benefits for Hair

When you incorporate peptides into your haircare routine, here's what you can expect:

1. ***Thicker, Fuller Hair***: By stimulating dormant hair follicles, peptides encourage regrowth and boost overall hair volume.
2. ***Reduced Hair Breakage***: Peptides strengthen the hair strand from the root, making them less likely to snap or split.
3. ***Scalp Nourishment***: A happy scalp is the secret to healthy hair. Peptides improve hydration and reduce inflammation, keeping your scalp balanced and nourished.

Peptides for Stronger Nails

Hair isn't the only thing that benefits from peptides. Brittle, peeling nails? Peptides can help! Just like with skin and hair, peptides play a role in boosting keratin production, the protein responsible for nail structure and strength.

One standout peptide for nail health is palmitoyl tripeptide-5. This peptide works by helping your body produce collagen, which in turn supports healthier nail beds and promotes faster nail growth. With consistent use in treatments or creams, it can help you grow stronger, shinier nails and prevent breakage.

Nail Benefits

The benefits of incorporating peptides into your nail care routine include:

1. ***Stronger Nail Plates***: Peptides improve keratin production, helping your nails withstand daily wear and tear.
2. ***Reduced Breakage***: If your nails tend to split or peel, peptides can strengthen them, reducing issues with fragility.
3. ***Faster Growth***: By encouraging healthier nail beds, peptides support quicker nail growth, so you can achieve long, beautiful nails with ease.

How to Incorporate Peptides Into Your Routine

Adding peptides to your hair and nail care regimen is easier than you think! Look for scalp serums, leave-in treatments, or conditioners formulated with peptides like copper peptides or acetyl tetrapeptide-3. For your nails, opt for strengthening creams or oils enriched with peptides to massage into your cuticles or nails.

With peptides working behind the scenes, you can say hello to thicker hair, fewer split ends, stronger nails, and less breakage. It's all about providing the essential building blocks your body needs to flourish.

Peptides are no longer just for your skin. They're an all-in-one solution for boosting hair growth and strengthening nails, helping you look and feel your best from head to toe. By improving follicle health for your hair and keratin production for your nails, these little molecules pack a big punch. Whether it's fuller, hydrated hair you're after or resilient, longer nails, peptides make for a smart addition to your routine.

Peptides for Longevity, Energy & Mood – Staying Vibrant at Any Age

In addition to improving the health and appearance of our skin, hair, and nails, peptides offer a range of benefits for overall wellness. Many peptides have been shown to increase longevity, boost energy levels, and enhance mood.

How Peptides Enhance Cellular Regeneration & Energy Levels

Peptides are like the body's tiny helpers, working behind the scenes to keep things running smoothly. One of their most impressive roles is in cellular regeneration, which is key to staying energetic and vibrant as we age. Every cell in the body has a lifespan—it gets worn out, replaced, or repaired. Peptides improve the speed and quality of this process, helping the body heal and renew itself from the inside out.

Specific peptides, like MOTS-c, play a significant role in optimizing how cells produce energy. Energy comes from mitochondria, often called the "powerhouses" of cells. Over time, mitochondrial function can decline, making you feel tired or less vibrant. Peptides that target mitochondria help reignite their energy production, making you feel more alert, active, and alive.

Additionally, peptides can reduce oxidative stress and inflammation, both of which cause damage over time. By supporting cellular repair and boosting the body's resilience, peptides help maintain the vitality needed for an active, healthy life at any age.

Brain-Boosting Peptides for Focus, Memory & Mood

Peptides are more than just skin and hair saviors; they also have incredible benefits for brain health. By enhancing focus, supporting memory, and improving mood, certain peptides are paving the way for sharper minds and happier lives. Two standout examples in this field are Semax and Dihexa, which have become popular tools for supporting cognitive function.

How Peptides Support Brain Health

The brain is a complex organ that thrives on communication. Neurons, the cells that make up the brain and nervous system, rely on chemical signals to stay connected and perform critical functions like memory, focus, and emotional regulation. Over time, or due to stress and other factors, these connections can weaken. This can lead to brain fog, difficulty concentrating, or even mood swings.

Peptides like Semax and Dihexa work to repair and strengthen these connections, making the brain sharper and more resilient. They're often referred to as nootropics, or "smart drugs," because of their ability to enhance mental performance. Unlike stimulants that only give a temporary boost, these peptides work at a deeper level, targeting the brain's natural ability to grow and adapt.

Semax: The Focus & Mood Enhancer

Semax is a neuropeptide with an impressive track record for supporting cognitive health. Originally developed in Russia for medical purposes, it's widely used for its ability to improve focus, memory, and mood.

How Semax Works

Semax boosts levels of brain-derived neurotrophic factor (BDNF), a type of protein that helps neurons grow and stay connected. Higher BDNF levels are linked to improved learning and memory because they foster the creation of new neural pathways.

Semax also influences the dopamine and serotonin systems in the brain. These chemicals are responsible for motivation and mood, respectively. By balancing these systems, Semax helps users feel focused, calm, and motivated.

Potential Benefits

1. Improved Focus: Semax enhances attention and concentration, making it easier to stay productive.
2. Memory Support: By promoting neural growth and connection, Semax aids in retaining information and recalling it when needed.
3. Mood Regulation: It positively impacts serotonin levels, which can lead to reduced stress and a more balanced mood.

Dihexa: The Memory Builder

Dihexa, another potent brain-boosting peptide, is often called a "brain repair" molecule. It's known for its impressive ability to strengthen existing neural pathways and even create new ones. For people looking to enhance long-term memory and brain resilience, Dihexa is an exciting candidate.

How Dihexa Works

Unlike many other nootropics, Dihexa directly binds to and activates specific receptors crucial for brain cell communication. This action promotes synaptogenesis, the process by which neurons form and strengthen their connections. This means Dihexa not only supports current brain function but also contributes to lasting improvements in memory and learning.

Potential Benefits

1. Enhanced Memory: Dihexa's ability to repair and create neural connections makes it particularly useful for improving memory retention and recall.
2. Neuroprotection: It may protect the brain from age-related decline by supporting overall brain health and function.
3. Supports Complex Thinking: By optimizing communication between neurons, Dihexa can enhance problem-solving and creative thinking.

Additional Benefits of Brain-Boosting Peptides

Beyond what Semax and Dihexa offer individually, peptides provide general benefits for brain health that can be life-changing. They combat oxidative stress, a major contributor to cognitive decline, by supporting the brain's natural repair processes. Peptides can also improve blood flow to the brain, ensuring it gets the oxygen and nutrients it needs to stay sharp.

It's important to emphasize that, while peptides show significant promise, their use should always be approached thoughtfully and under the guidance of a healthcare professional. With ongoing research and developments, the potential for peptides in brain health continues to grow, giving people new ways to optimize their mental performance and overall well-being.

Brain health is central to everything we do. Whether it's staying on top of daily tasks, learning new skills, or simply feeling happy and motivated, peptides offer a way to support the brain's incredible capabilities over a lifetime.

Peptides for Sleep & Stress Relief to Combat Burnout

Burnout has become a widespread issue, impacting people's health and productivity alike. The combination of chronic stress and poor sleep creates a vicious cycle that makes recovery feel out of reach.

Fortunately, peptides offer a promising approach to tackling both stress and sleep issues, helping individuals regain their energy, focus, and overall resilience. Peptides like Epitalon and Selank stand out for their restorative benefits, addressing the root causes of sleepless nights and high stress without the drawbacks of traditional medications.

Peptides for Sleep Support

Sleep is essential for physical and mental recovery, but it's often the first casualty of a demanding lifestyle. Many people struggle with falling asleep, staying asleep, or achieving the deep, restorative rest that the body and brain need. This is where peptides like Epitalon come into play, offering support by enhancing the body's natural sleep regulation systems.

How Epitalon Works

Epitalon is a peptide that regulates melatonin, the hormone responsible for controlling the sleep-wake cycle. Melatonin production often decreases with age, travel, or exposure to stressors, disrupting the body's internal clock. By supporting melatonin release, Epitalon helps reset this clock, making it easier to fall asleep consistently and wake up refreshed.

But the benefits of Epitalon extend beyond sleep regulation. It is also believed to enhance the quality of sleep by promoting deep, restorative phases essential for body repair and brain function. Deep sleep is when the body clears toxins from the brain, repairs tissues, and restores energy. When Epitalon helps users achieve better sleep, it contributes to improved mental clarity, emotional balance, and physical endurance.

Benefits of Epitalon for Sleep

1. *Improved Sleep-Wake Cycle*: Epitalon helps establish a steady circadian rhythm, so you fall asleep and wake up at consistent times.
2. *Enhanced Restorative Sleep*: It fosters deeper sleep stages, crucial for brain health and energy recovery.
3. *Support for Long-Term Resilience*: Better sleep builds a foundation for combating stress, improving mood, and maintaining energy levels over time.

Peptides for Stress Relief

Chronic stress is a significant driver of burnout. It triggers the body's fight-or-flight response, flooding it with stress hormones like cortisol. While this is helpful in short bursts, prolonged stress leaves you feeling drained, overwhelmed, or emotionally unstable. Peptides like Selank provide an innovative way to reduce stress without causing unwanted side effects like grogginess or dependence.

How Selank Works

Selank is a peptide that interacts with neurotransmitters in the brain, particularly those associated with anxiety and mood regulation. It enhances the stability of these chemical systems, helping to reduce overactivity in the stress-response pathways. Unlike many anti-anxiety medications, Selank doesn't act as a sedative. Instead, it promotes a sense of calm by addressing overexcited neural responses at their source.

Selank also supports cognitive function under stress. Stress often leads to "brain fog," making it harder to focus or problem-solve effectively. By calming the nervous system, Selank allows the brain to work more efficiently, whether you're handling a high-pressure project or simply trying to unwind after a tough day.

<u>Benefits of Selank for Stress Management</u>

1. *Reduced Anxiety Levels*: Selank lowers feelings of worry and overstimulation, making daily stressors easier to handle.

2. ***Enhanced Emotional Balance***: It stabilizes mood without causing sedation or grogginess like traditional stress-relief drugs.
3. ***Better Focus Under Pressure***: By calming the mind, Selank helps preserve mental clarity and cognitive performance, even in stressful situations.

By addressing two of the main contributors to burnout—poor sleep and chronic stress—Epitalon and Selank provide a dual approach that fosters recovery and resilience. Better sleep through Epitalon allows the body to recover its energy stores and repair physical and mental damage. At the same time, stress reduction through Selank lowers cortisol levels and provides emotional relief, preventing the chronic tension that leads to burnout.

This combination creates a positive feedback loop. Improved sleep enhances your tolerance for stress, while reduced stress creates the conditions needed for better sleep. Together, these peptides offer profound support for individuals looking to break free from the cycle of exhaustion and regain control over their well-being.

Peptides like Epitalon and Selank represent a new frontier in combating the physical and mental toll of modern life. They go beyond masking symptoms, addressing underlying issues that disrupt sleep and heighten stress. With regular use, these peptides can help restore balance, improve mental clarity, and support physical resilience, all while promoting a greater sense of calm and relaxation.

However, like any supplement, the use of peptides should be carefully considered and guided by a healthcare professional. When paired with other self-care practices like proper nutrition, regular exercise, and mindfulness, peptides can be a valuable tool in overcoming burnout and achieving a healthier, more balanced life.

How to Safely Get Started – Sourcing, Dosage & Legal Considerations

Peptides can offer incredible benefits when used correctly. But like anything that affects your body, safety is key. Before jumping in, it's essential to understand where to source peptides, how to use them properly, and how to monitor your results. This chapter covers the basics to help you get started confidently and responsibly.

Understanding Peptide Regulations & Safe Sourcing for Women

Peptides may sound like a miracle solution, but they aren't regulated the same way as prescription medications. This makes it important to do your research when selecting a supplier. Here are some tips for sourcing peptides safely:

1. ***Know the Legal Status in Your Country***: Laws surrounding peptides vary depending on where you live. Some countries allow peptides for research purposes only, while others permit personal use as long

as they're sourced responsibly. Take the time to familiarize yourself with your local regulations, as this can help you avoid legal issues.

2. **Find a Reputable Vendor**: Not all peptide suppliers are created equal. Look for companies that offer transparency about their products, including third-party testing for purity and quality. Reviews from other users can also give you insight into trustworthy sources. Avoid sketchy websites or offers that sound too good to be true.

3. **Consult a Medical Professional**: Before buying or using peptides, talk to a qualified healthcare provider. Professionals familiar with peptides can guide you on where to source them safely and which options are best for your needs. This is especially important for women since hormonal balances may affect how your body responds to peptides.

By understanding peptide regulations and sourcing from reputable vendors, you can prioritize safety and effectiveness. Always consult a healthcare professional to ensure peptides are right for you and your specific needs.

How to Dose Peptides for Maximum Benefits with Minimal Risk

Once you've sourced your peptides, the next step is understanding dosing. Getting this right is essential to avoid side effects and make the most of their benefits.

1. **Start Low and Go Slow**: It's tempting to jump in with high doses to see results quickly, but this can backfire. Starting with a lower dose gives your body time to adjust and reduces the risk of side effects. For example, with peptides like BPC-157 or MOTS-c, start with a dose at the lower end of the recommended range and gradually increase as needed.
2. **Follow Manufacturer or Physician Guidelines**: When dosing peptides, always follow the instructions provided by the supplier or your healthcare provider. Every peptide is different, so there is no one-size-fits-all approach. Factors like your weight, age, and medical history may influence your ideal dosage.
3. **Injectables vs. Topicals vs. Oral Peptides**: Peptides come in various forms, including injectables, creams, and oral capsules. Injectable peptides are typically the most effective because they bypass digestion and get straight to work in the body. If you're using injectable peptides, make sure you're trained on sterile techniques to minimize the risk of infection.

4. ***Track How Your Body Responds***: Keep a journal to track your progress. Note down how you're feeling, any noticeable changes, and whether you're experiencing side effects. This information can help you and your healthcare provider make adjustments as needed.

Dosing peptides correctly is key to maximizing their benefits while minimizing risks. Always start low, follow professional guidance, and monitor your body's response to ensure safe and effective results.

When to Cycle Peptides & How to Monitor Your Progress

Peptides have gained popularity for their wide-ranging health benefits, from enhancing energy levels to improving skin health. However, using peptides effectively involves more than simply starting and continuing indefinitely.

Like many wellness solutions, peptides must be used strategically to ensure their benefits remain consistent and sustainable. This process, known as cycling, is vital for maximizing their effectiveness while minimizing potential risks.

Why Cycling Peptides is Essential

Cycling refers to using peptides for a specific period, followed by a break. This approach prevents two major concerns that can arise from continuous use:

1. **Reduced Effectiveness**: The body can become desensitized to certain peptides when they are consistently used over time. Cycling allows your cells and receptors to reset, maintaining the peptides' potency during subsequent cycles.
2. **Risk of Overstimulation**: Peptides often work by activating specific biological pathways. Prolonged use without breaks can overstimulate these pathways, potentially leading to imbalances or unwanted side effects. Rest periods allow the body to recalibrate.

By adhering to a cyclical approach, users can enjoy consistent, sustainable benefits while reducing the likelihood of complications.

Typical Peptide Cycle Durations

Most peptides are used in cycles ranging from 4 to 12 weeks, depending on the type of peptide, its purpose, and individual goals. The break period following a cycle is equally important, typically lasting as long as or longer than the cycle itself. Here are a few examples to illustrate how cycling works for different peptides:

1. ***Growth Hormone-Releasing Peptides (e.g., CJC-1295 with Ipamorelin)***: These peptides stimulate growth hormone production, promoting fat metabolism, muscle recovery, and better sleep. A common cycle lasts 8 to 12 weeks, followed by a break of the same duration. Cycling ensures the body doesn't develop resistance and continues to respond optimally.
2. ***Skin-Repair Peptides (e.g., GHK-Cu)***: These peptides are often used for specific needs, such as accelerating wound healing or improving skin elasticity. Their cycles might be shorter, typically 4 to 6 weeks, depending on the desired outcome. After achieving results, users may pause to monitor the skin's progress without continual input.
3. ***Metabolism-Enhancing Peptides (e.g., MOTS-c)***: Since these peptides target mitochondrial function and energy levels, cycles often last 6 to 10 weeks, followed by a break to ensure the body recalibrates and avoids overstimulation.

Ultimately, cycle lengths should be tailored to individual goals and responses. Consulting a healthcare provider can help determine the optimal duration for both use and rest periods.

How to Monitor Your Progress

Tracking progress during peptide use is crucial for understanding their effectiveness and ensuring that they align with your health and wellness goals. Monitoring can be broken into two categories:

Objective Measures

1. *Physical Changes*: Track metrics like body weight, body fat percentage, muscle mass, or specific skin improvements (e.g., reduced wrinkles, improved texture).
2. *Lab Tests*: Regular blood work can assess hormone levels, inflammatory markers, or other relevant parameters associated with the peptide's benefits. For example, growth hormone levels can be monitored when using CJC-1295, while GHK-Cu's effects might show in improved collagen biomarkers.
3. *Performance Metrics*: If the peptide targets physical performance or energy, measure outcomes such as stamina during exercise or recovery time after workouts.

Subjective Measures

1. *Mood and Mental Clarity*: Note any improvements in mental sharpness, focus, or emotional well-being. For instance, peptides like Selank, known for stress relief, can make a noticeable difference in mood stability.
2. *Energy Levels*: Keep track of how energized you feel throughout the day.

3. ***Quality of Sleep***: Since peptides often enhance sleep patterns, record how rested you feel upon waking, or consider using sleep trackers for more detailed insights.

Maintaining a journal or app to document these observations can reveal trends over the course of a peptide cycle.

Reassessing Before Starting a New Cycle

Before beginning a new peptide cycle, take time to evaluate whether your goals were met. Consider these steps to reassess:

1. ***Review Results***: Compare your tracking data to your initial goals. For example, did CJC-1295 improve your energy and metabolism as expected? Did your skin benefit from GHK-Cu?
2. ***Adjust Goals if Needed***: If the peptide met your expectations, you might not need another cycle immediately. If results were inconsistent, consult with your healthcare provider to discuss alternative dosing strategies, peptide combinations, or lifestyle changes that could enhance results.
3. ***Plan for Sustainability***: Consider how peptides fit into your overall wellness plan. They should complement healthy behaviors, such as a balanced diet, exercise,

and stress management, rather than act as standalone solutions.

Watch for Side Effects

Although peptides are generally well-tolerated, side effects can occur, especially with improper use. Recognizing and addressing these issues early ensures safe and effective cycling. Common side effects include:

- *Mild Nausea or Headaches*: These symptoms might occur as the body adjusts to peptides.
- *Injection Site Irritation*: Redness, swelling, or discomfort may arise if injectable peptides are not administered properly.
- *Unintended Hormonal Effects*: Overuse or misuse of peptides like those affecting growth hormone pathways may lead to imbalances.

If you experience any persistent or concerning symptoms, pause peptide use immediately and consult your healthcare provider. This step is crucial for preventing complications and ensuring that your peptide protocol aligns with your personal health profile.

Starting your peptide journey doesn't have to be intimidating. By understanding regulations, sourcing peptides safely, dosing them correctly, and monitoring your progress, you can maximize the benefits while minimizing risks.

Remember, peptides aren't a quick fix—they're a tool to support a healthier, more vibrant physique and mindset. With the right information and guidance, you'll be well on your way to unlocking their potential!

The 3-Week Peptide Protocol for Women's Wellness

Women's bodies have unique needs and sensitivities, which is why a specific peptide protocol tailored for women's wellness can be highly beneficial. The following 3-week protocol is designed to address common concerns such as skin aging, hormonal imbalances, and stress management.

Week 1: Detailed Plan – Hormonal Reset & Energy Boost

This week sets the foundation for balancing your hormones and optimizing your energy. By using CJC-1295 with Ipamorelin, you'll encourage your body to naturally boost growth hormone levels, which can benefit hormone regulation, sleep, recovery, and metabolism. Pair the peptide with supportive nutrition, exercise, and self-care practices to maximize results.

Day 1

- *Peptide Plan*: Take your first dose of CJC-1295 with Ipamorelin as a subcutaneous injection in the evening

before bed. Start with the recommended low dose, as this complements your natural nightly release of growth hormone.
- ***Diet Tips***: Focus on healthy fats like avocado, olive oil, or nuts. Prepare balanced meals with lean protein (like grilled chicken or tofu) and lots of greens to support hormone function.
- ***Exercise***: Start your week with light exercise, like a brisk 20-minute walk, stretching, or gentle yoga.
- ***Self-Care***: Create an evening routine to prepare your body for deep sleep. This might include dim lighting, a cup of chamomile tea, and journaling your intentions for the week.

Day 2

- ***Peptide Plan***: Administer your next dose of CJC-1295 with Ipamorelin at bedtime, sticking to a roughly consistent time each evening.
- ***Diet Tips***: Hydration is key! Drink at least 8–10 glasses of water throughout the day. Add zinc-rich foods like spinach or pumpkin seeds to your meals to optimize hormone production.
- ***Exercise***: Incorporate 15 minutes of gentle yoga or Pilates. Focus on stretches that activate the core and relieve tension.

- *Self-Care*: Try 5–10 minutes of deep breathing or mindfulness meditation before bed to lower cortisol (stress hormone) levels.

Day 3

- *Peptide Plan*: Continue your bedtime CJC-1295 dose to enhance your body's repair and rejuvenation during sleep.
- *Diet Tips*: Swap out processed snacks for natural options like a handful of almonds or apple slices with nut butter. Pair your lunch with a side of fermented foods (like kimchi or yogurt) to support gut health, which is closely tied to hormone balance.
- *Exercise*: Introduce light strength training today—bodyweight exercises like squats and push-ups are a great starting point. Aim for 15–20 minutes.
- *Self-Care*: Take note of any small changes in your energy levels or mood. Journaling these observations can help you track progress and tweak your routine.

Day 4

- *Peptide Plan*: Administer your fourth dose of CJC-1295 with Ipamorelin in the evening. Consistency ensures the peptides build their effects over time.
- *Diet Tips*: Include omega-3-rich foods like salmon, chia seeds, or flaxseeds to combat inflammation and support hormone health.

- *Exercise*: Go for a 25-minute power walk or do a light jog to boost your metabolism and improve circulation.
- *Self-Care*: Enjoy a 15-minute Epsom salt bath in the evening to relax your muscles and promote recovery from exercise.

Day 5

- *Peptide Plan*: Take your final CJC-1295 dose of the week before bed. The weekend will act as a rest period for the peptide.
- *Diet Tips*: Prioritize protein at every meal – eggs for breakfast, lean turkey for lunch, and grilled fish for dinner. Protein helps repair muscles and balances hunger hormones like ghrelin.
- *Exercise*: Engage in light resistance exercises, focusing on building lean muscle. Use dumbbells or resistance bands if you have them.
- *Self-Care*: Reward yourself for the week's consistency with a low-sugar dark chocolate treat or an extra 30 minutes of "you time."

Day 6

- *Peptide Plan*: No peptides today; allow your body to rest and reset.
- *Diet Tips*: Start your day with a nutrient-packed smoothie using spinach, frozen berries, almond butter, and a scoop of collagen or protein powder.

- *Exercise*: Choose a low-impact activity you enjoy, like hiking or dancing. Moving for 30 minutes will help sustain the momentum.
- *Self-Care*: Schedule time for a hobby or activity that brings you joy. This is your reward for staying committed during the week.

Day 7

- *Peptide Plan*: Rest day for peptides, giving your body time to process and adapt.
- *Diet Tips*: Focus on fiber-rich meals to support digestion and hormonal detox. Add vegetables like broccoli, kale, or Brussels sprouts to your plate.
- *Exercise*: Try a restorative yoga session or simple stretching to improve flexibility and prepare your mind and body for the upcoming week.
- *Self-Care*: Reflect on how you feel after one week of the protocol. Celebrate small wins, like better sleep or improved mood, and plan your Week 2 goals.

By the end of Week 1, you'll have set a strong foundation for hormonal balance and energy enhancement. While immediate results may vary, you should start to notice improved sleep, steady energy levels, and perhaps a calmer mindset. Stick with the protocol, as Week 2 brings even more exciting benefits!

Week 2: Detailed Plan – Skin Rejuvenation & Fat Loss Acceleration

This week is all about enhancing your skin's radiance and tackling stubborn fat. Peptides like GHK-Cu supercharge collagen production for firmer, glowing skin, while Tesamorelin helps break down abdominal fat and preserve lean muscle. Combine these with supportive diet, exercise, and self-care for visible results.

Day 8

- *Peptide Plan*: Administer Tesamorelin via a subcutaneous injection in the morning to activate fat metabolism. Apply GHK-Cu peptide serum to your skin in the evening after cleansing.
- *Diet Tips*: Focus on an antioxidant-rich diet today. Add blueberries, almonds, and dark leafy greens to your meals to repair and protect your skin.
- *Exercise*: Start your day with a 10-minute warm-up, then incorporate resistance training to build lean muscle. Try squats, lunges, or push-ups for 20 minutes.
- *Self-Care*: Gently exfoliate your skin during your nighttime routine for better absorption of the GHK-Cu serum, and hydrate well before bed.

Day 9

- *Peptide Plan*: Administer your Tesamorelin dose in the morning and reapply GHK-Cu serum before bed.

- ***Diet Tips***: Include salmon or other omega-3-rich foods at lunch to reduce inflammation and improve skin elasticity. Pair with whole grains like quinoa for sustained energy.
- ***Exercise***: Focus on interval training—alternate between brisk walking or running for 1 minute and a slower pace for 2 minutes. Repeat for 20–30 minutes.
- ***Self-Care***: Moisturize your skin twice today to keep it hydrated and amplify the effects of GHK-Cu. Add sunscreen if you're heading outdoors, as your skin may be extra sensitive.

Day 10

- ***Peptide Plan***: Continue with your morning Tesamorelin dose and the GHK-Cu serum at night. Be consistent with the timing of both peptides for optimal results.
- ***Diet Tips***: Boost collagen production with bone broth or a collagen supplement. Add vitamin C-rich foods like oranges or bell peppers to help your body process collagen effectively.
- ***Exercise***: Focus on strength exercises targeting your upper body (shoulder presses, rows) to support muscle-building efforts. Dedicate 20–25 minutes.
- ***Self-Care***: Pamper your skin by adding a hydrating sheet mask after applying GHK-Cu. Use this time to unwind and relax.

Day 11

- *Peptide Plan*: After your morning Tesamorelin injection, ensure you stay hydrated throughout the day to maximize fat-loss effects. Apply GHK-Cu serum before bed.
- *Diet Tips*: Snack on healthy fats like walnuts or avocado. Include a protein-rich dinner with chicken or tofu to help maintain lean muscle mass.
- *Exercise*: Take a brisk 30-minute walk to stay active, followed by stretching to improve flexibility and circulation.
- *Self-Care*: Practice 10 minutes of mindfulness or meditation to de-stress, as cortisol can impact both fat loss and skin health.

Day 12

- *Peptide Plan*: Final day of the peptide cycle for the week—take your Tesamorelin dose in the morning and use GHK-Cu at night. Allow your body to rest over the weekend.
- *Diet Tips*: Eliminate processed carbs today. Instead, fuel your day with quinoa or sweet potatoes, paired with green vegetables and lean proteins.
- *Exercise*: Do a HIIT (High-Intensity Interval Training) session focusing on lower-body exercises. Aim for 20–25 minutes.

- *Self-Care*: Treat yourself to a facial massage during your evening skincare routine. It improves circulation and enhances collagen production.

Day 13

- *Peptide Plan*: Rest day for both Tesamorelin and GHK-Cu peptides. Use this break to allow your body to reset and adapt.
- *Diet Tips*: Start your morning with a nourishing smoothie (spinach, frozen berries, almond milk, and a scoop of protein or collagen powder).
- *Exercise*: Spend time outdoors for a light activity like a nature walk or bike ride. Aim for 30–40 minutes to promote mental clarity and physical recovery.
- *Self-Care*: Dedicate part of your day to hobbies or leisure activities that make you happy—this helps reduce stress and keeps your hormones balanced.

Day 14

- *Peptide Plan*: Another rest day for peptides. Keep your skin hydrated with your usual moisturizer, and avoid harsh skincare treatments.
- *Diet Tips*: Focus on anti-inflammatory foods such as turmeric tea, ginger, and green tea. Pair them with whole, nutrient-dense meals.

- *Exercise*: Finish the week with a restorative yoga session or simple stretches to prepare for your Week 3 transition.
- *Self-Care*: Reflect on this week's results—take note of changes in your skin's texture or fat loss progress. Use this reflection to refine your goals going forward.

By the end of Week 2, with consistency in using Tesamorelin and GHK-Cu, you may start noticing subtle improvements in your skin's appearance and a reduction in stubborn fat. The combination of peptides, nutrition, and exercise is powering your transformation—keep building on this momentum as you prepare for Week 3!

Week 3: Detailed Plan – Longevity & Anti-Aging Optimization

This final week focuses on promoting long-term health, cellular repair, and mental clarity. By using peptides like Epitalon and Semax, you'll support anti-aging at a cellular level while sharpening your cognitive function. Pair this with holistic habits such as mindful eating and restorative activities to finish your wellness protocol feeling radiant and empowered.

Day 15

- *Peptide Plan*: Take Epitalon as a subcutaneous injection in the morning to activate cellular repair and promote longevity. Use Semax as a nasal spray earlier in the day to boost mental clarity and focus.

- *Diet Tips*: Start your morning with a cup of green tea and walnuts for their anti-aging antioxidants and healthy fats. Include colorful veggies like bell peppers and carrots in your meals for skin-boosting vitamins.
- *Exercise*: Do a 20-minute low-impact cardio routine, such as cycling or dancing, to engage your body without overloading it.
- *Self-Care*: Write down your long-term health goals. Reflect on how each step of this protocol supports your vision for aging gracefully.

Day 16

- *Peptide Plan*: Administer your Epitalon injection in the morning and take another dose of Semax for enhanced focus and memory support.
- *Diet Tips*: Add cruciferous vegetables like broccoli or cauliflower to your meals. These foods help reduce inflammation and oxidative stress, which speeds up aging.
- *Exercise*: Try a brisk 30-minute outdoor walk. The sunlight and fresh air can improve your mood and energy levels.
- *Self-Care*: Dedicate 10 minutes to mindfulness meditation or breathing exercises to reduce stress, which can accelerate aging.

Day 17

- *Peptide Plan*: Continue the same dosage of Epitalon in the morning and Semax as needed for mental and mood enhancement.
- *Diet Tips*: Sip on turmeric tea, which is rich in anti-inflammatory compounds, and include a serving of lean protein with every meal to aid cellular repair.
- *Exercise*: Do strength-training exercises for 15–20 minutes to maintain bone density and build lean muscle mass. Focus on functional movements like squats and deadlifts.
- *Self-Care*: Treat yourself to a rejuvenating skincare routine, such as a calming face mask rich in antioxidants, to care for your external glow as well.

Day 18

- *Peptide Plan*: Administer Epitalon in the morning and Semax during mid-morning. Stay consistent with your doses to build optimal results.
- *Diet Tips*: Include healthy fats like avocado and fatty fish such as salmon in your meals. These fats promote cellular membrane health and improve skin elasticity.
- *Exercise*: Stretch or foam roll for 15–20 minutes to increase blood flow, improve flexibility, and reduce tension.
- *Self-Care*: Journal your feelings of gratitude and reflect on the positive changes you've experienced

during the protocol. A positive mindset supports longevity and well-being.

Day 19

- *Peptide Plan*: Take Epitalon in the morning and a dose of Semax if you'd like a mental clarity boost.
- *Diet Tips*: Snack on antioxidant-rich dark chocolate or green tea to support your body's defense against free radicals. Keep your meals protein-forward with some leafy greens on the side.
- *Exercise*: Focus on moderate-intensity cardio, like a 30-minute jog or incline walking, to keep your heart healthy.
- *Self-Care*: Unwind with an evening guided meditation or light a calming scented candle to prepare for deep, restorative sleep.

Day 20

- *Peptide Plan*: Continue taking both Epitalon (morning) and Semax (mid-morning or before a mentally demanding activity).
- *Diet Tips*: Incorporate fermented foods like sauerkraut or yogurt into your meals to support gut health and a strong immune system.
- *Exercise*: Take part in an enjoyable physical activity, like swimming or a dance class. Movement is medicine, so keep it fun and engaging.

- *Self-Care*: Treat yourself to time outdoors, whether relaxing in a garden, walking through a park, or enjoying a quiet picnic. Fresh air replenishes your mental energy.

Day 21

- *Peptide Plan*: Take your final doses of Epitalon in the morning to conclude the peptide protocol. Use Semax earlier in the day as a finishing touch to mental clarity and focus.
- *Diet Tips*: Round out your dietary week with a nutrient-dense meal filled with vibrant veggies, lean protein, and healthy fats. Sip on chamomile tea after dinner to aid digestion.
- *Exercise*: Wrap up the week with a restorative yoga session or slow stretching routine to relax your body and mind.
- *Self-Care*: Reflect on your 3-week progress. Write down what changes you've seen and your plan for sustaining these results going forward. Celebrate your commitment to your health and longevity!

By the end of Week 3, you'll have taken major strides in promoting cellular repair, improving mental clarity, and reducing the effects of aging. Remember, this is only the beginning of a long-term wellness story—you've built a foundation for staying vibrant and strong for years to come! Keep refining your self-care regimen and cycling peptides when needed to continue reaping the rewards.

Troubleshooting & Adjusting for Your Unique Body

Your wellness journey is personal, and your body may respond differently to peptides than others'. This chapter is your roadmap to manage side effects, adjust dosages, and overcome challenges, especially if you don't see the results you hoped for. You'll also learn how to maintain your progress and cycle peptides safely for long-term benefits.

Recognizing Common Side Effects

It's normal to experience minor adjustments as your body adapts, but it's crucial to distinguish between harmless effects and those that need attention. Here are some common side effects and what they may mean for you:

1. **Injection Site Reactions**

   What to Expect: Redness, swelling, or itching at the injection site. This is usually mild and temporary.

   What to Do:

- Ensure you're using sterile equipment and proper injection techniques.
- Apply a cold compress to reduce redness or swelling.
- Rotate injection sites to avoid irritation in one area.

2. **Temporary Fatigue or Brain Fog**

What to Expect: Some peptides, like CJC-1295, can initially cause fatigue as your body adjusts to increased growth hormone activity.

What to Do:

- Stay hydrated and ensure you're getting adequate rest.
- If fatigue persists, consider reducing your dosage slightly and monitoring how you feel.

3. **Mild Headaches**

What to Expect: Semax, for example, may sometimes cause headaches in sensitive individuals.

What to Do:

- Drink plenty of water and take breaks from mentally demanding tasks.
- If the issue continues, reduce Semax usage or space out doses more widely during the day.

4. **Skin Tightness or Sensitivity**

   What to Expect: GHK-Cu can make your skin feel tighter or more sensitive as it boosts collagen production.

   What to Do:

   - Use gentle, hydrating skincare products and apply sunscreen daily.
   - Cut back on exfoliation or other abrasive treatments until your skin adjusts.

5. **Nausea or Digestive Discomfort**

   What to Expect: Some peptides, like Tesamorelin, may cause slight nausea when starting.

   What to Do:

   - Take peptides on an empty stomach to improve absorption if nausea occurs.
   - If it persists, try a smaller dose and gradually increase it over time.
   - If any side effects are severe or persist beyond a few days, stop the peptide and consult with a healthcare professional before continuing.

When to Adjust Dosages

Your body's needs may change throughout the protocol. Adjusting the dosage is a helpful way to dial in the benefits while minimizing side effects. Here's how to approach dosage changes safely:

1. **Start Low and Taper Up**
   - Always begin with the lowest recommended dose for the peptide you're using.
   - Over 2–3 weeks, gradually increase the dose (if needed), monitoring how your body responds.

   Example: With CJC-1295, start with a small dose (say, 200mcg) and increase by 50mcg weekly if you're tolerating it well but not seeing results.

2. **Reduce Dosage Temporarily**
   - If you experience side effects like fatigue or nausea, reduce the dosage by 20–30% for a few days.
   - Track how you feel—if symptoms improve, maintain the lower dose or slowly work your way back up.

3. **Take Rest Periods**
   - Some peptides, like Tesamorelin, can lose effectiveness if the body becomes resistant to them.
   - Incorporate rest days (weekend breaks, for example), or take a longer pause for a few weeks as needed.

4. **Adjust Timing of Doses**
    - Some peptides may work better at specific times of the day. For example, take CJC-1295 with Ipamorelin in the evening to align with your body's natural growth hormone release.
    - If a peptide causes daytime fatigue, try shifting the dose to later hours or during a rest period.

Keeping a journal of your dosing schedule, side effects, and benefits can help you identify patterns and decide when adjustments are needed.

When to Consult a Healthcare Professional

You know your body better than anyone, but there are times when expert guidance is essential. Reach out to a healthcare provider if you experience any of the following:

- Persistent or severe side effects (e.g., intense headaches, prolonged nausea or swelling, mood changes).
- Symptoms that interfere with your daily life or overall wellness.
- Uncertainty about the correct dosage or administration method.
- An underlying condition that may be impacted by peptides (e.g., thyroid, autoimmune, or metabolic disorders).

Your healthcare provider can suggest lab tests to track markers like hormone levels, inflammation, or cellular aging, helping you tailor the protocol to suit your needs.

What to Do If You Don't See Results – Common Pitfalls & Fixes

Sometimes, despite your best efforts, progress may feel slower than expected. Here's how you can troubleshoot and make meaningful adjustments to get back on track.

1. **Evaluate Dosage and Administration**
   - **Pitfall:** You might be using too little or too much of a peptide, or the timing might be incorrect.
   - **Fix:** Revisit your protocol and ensure you're following the recommended dosage. Start with the lowest dose and gradually increase only if needed. For example, if you're using CJC-1295 with Ipamorelin, confirm your timing aligns with natural circadian hormone rhythms (evening dosing is best).
   - **Tip:** Double-check your injection technique to ensure proper absorption of subcutaneous peptides. If you're unsure, consult a healthcare provider.

2. **Stay Consistent**
   - **Pitfall:** Skipping doses or treating peptides as a "quick fix" without changes to diet or lifestyle can hinder results.
   - **Fix:** Commit to a schedule and set reminders to help you stick to it. Peptides work best when used consistently as part of a holistic approach, so pair them with supportive habits like nutritious meals, regular exercise, and sufficient sleep.
   - **Tip:** Create a weekly planner and block specific times for administering peptides and key self-care routines.
3. **Review Your Lifestyle Foundations**
   - **Pitfall:** Poor diet, lack of sleep, or chronic stress may blunt the effectiveness of peptides.
   - **Fix:** Focus on the basics.
   - **Nutrition:** Anti-inflammatory, nutrient-dense foods like fatty fish, leafy greens, and whole grains optimize peptide benefits.
   - **Sleep:** Ensure 7–8 hours of quality sleep to support recovery and peptide activity.
   - **Stress:** Practice relaxation techniques to minimize cortisol, which can counteract the effects of growth-promoting peptides.

4. **Adjust Expectations**
   - **Pitfall:** Unrealistic timelines for results can lead to frustration. Remember, changes like fat loss or improved skin elasticity take time and consistent effort.
   - **Fix:** Reflect on your goals and break them into smaller milestones. Track subtle changes—such as better sleep, improved energy, or plumper skin—to recognize progress.

5. **Assess the Peptide Protocol Appropriateness**
   - **Pitfall:** The peptide you're using may not align perfectly with your goals or body's needs.
   - **Fix:** Rotate or introduce complementary peptides. For example, if GHK-Cu isn't producing visible skin results, consider whether combining it with Tesamorelin for body composition improvements might amplify overall changes.
   - **Tip:** Speak to a professional to fine-tune your protocol, especially if you're addressing complex needs like hormonal imbalances.

6. **Monitor External Factors**
   - **Pitfall:** Environmental toxins, dehydration, or overtraining could counteract progress.
   - **Fix:** Stay hydrated (at least 2 liters of water daily), reduce toxin exposure, and balance your workouts with recovery days.

7. **Seek Professional Input**
   - **Pitfall:** Persistent lack of results may indicate underlying health issues like thyroid imbalance or insulin resistance.
   - **Fix:** Consult a healthcare provider to assess your baseline health and run relevant tests for advanced troubleshooting.

Achieving results with peptides takes consistency, the right protocol, and a holistic approach to health. By addressing common pitfalls and making targeted adjustments, you can maximize their effectiveness and stay on track toward your goals.

Long-Term Strategies: How to Maintain Benefits & Cycle Peptides Safely

Your 3-week protocol is designed to jumpstart your wellness, but sustainable health is a long-term commitment. These strategies will help you maintain your progress and integrate peptides into your lifestyle safely.

1. **Know When to Cycle Off**
   - Over time, your body can adapt to continuous peptide usage, reducing its effectiveness. Cycling peptides ensures your body remains responsive.
   - For most peptides (like **CJC-1295, Tesamorelin, or Epitalon**), experts recommend

taking at least 2–4 weeks off between cycles. For example:
- Use peptides for 3 months and then take at least one month off.
- Alternatively, follow a pattern like 5 days on and 2 days off weekly to build breaks directly into your protocol.
- Pay attention to your body—symptoms like plateauing results or heightened fatigue could signal it's time for a pause.

2. **Develop a Sustainable Routine**
   - ***Simplify Your Plan***: Overcomplicating your schedule can lead to burnout. Stick with key peptides for the most pressing concerns rather than adding too many at once.
   - ***Rotate Target Areas***: Want to focus on fat loss, skin health, and cognitive well-being? Make each a priority during different cycles instead of doing everything simultaneously.
   - ***Use Checkpoints***: Every 3–6 months, set aside time to revisit your goals. Evaluate if your current regimen aligns with your evolving needs.

3. **Monitor Your Health Over Time**
   - ***Track Progress Beyond the Mirror***: Look at your workout performance, mood stability,

recovery time, and overall vitality as markers of success.
- **Get Regular Checkups**: Blood tests for hormone levels, inflammation markers, or nutrient deficiencies can reveal deeper insights into how peptides are serving your body.

4. **Pair Peptides with Healthy Foundations**

Peptides amplify your body's natural potential, but they thrive on a solid foundation of healthy practices:

- *Diet*: Stick to clean, whole foods with plenty of healthy fats, lean proteins, and colorful vegetables.
- *Fitness*: Consistent strength training and low-impact cardio support muscle growth, metabolic health, and longevity.
- *Sleep Hygiene*: Deep, restorative sleep is non-negotiable for anti-aging and hormone repair. Create a bedtime ritual to optimize rest.

5. **Stay Curious and Evolve**
   - Science around peptides is constantly growing. Stay informed and open to exploring new compounds or protocols for emerging wellness goals.
   - Work with knowledgeable professionals who can tailor updates to your peptides based on cutting-edge research.

6. **Be Kind to Yourself**

    Long-term health doesn't mean perfection. Some cycles may bring dramatic improvements, others subtler shifts. Celebrate the progress you make and adjust when life throws curveballs. Wellness is a lifelong marathon, not a sprint.

By addressing common pitfalls, fine-tuning dosages, and committing to long-term strategies, you're setting yourself up for sustained health and vitality. The key is consistency, self-awareness, and a willingness to adapt as your body evolves. Through mindful use and strategic maintenance, peptides can remain an empowering tool for your lifelong wellness.

Conclusion

The possibilities of peptides in women's health are as exciting as they are empowering. This guide has walked you through the core principles of using peptides effectively, troubleshooting side effects, adjusting dosages, and maintaining long-term benefits. At the heart of it all is the understanding that your body is unique, and personalization is key.

By listening to your body, monitoring how it responds, and tailoring your peptide protocol to suit your specific needs, you can unlock incredible potential for your health and well-being.

But peptides are just one piece of the puzzle. Building a sustainable wellness routine that goes beyond peptides is essential for achieving lasting health. Focus on core pillars like nutrition, regular exercise, quality sleep, and stress management.

Pair these with mindfulness practices, like journaling, meditation, or spending time in nature, to nurture your mental and emotional well-being alongside the physical. Remember, it's about creating habits you can maintain—small, consistent actions often lead to the biggest changes over time.

To continue your learning and growth, equip yourself with reliable resources. Look for trusted websites, books, and online communities dedicated to health, wellness, and peptides. Seek out healthcare professionals who are knowledgeable about peptides and can provide personalized advice. Surround yourself with a supportive network of people who motivate and inspire you. Wellness is never a solo endeavor—connecting with others can make the process more dynamic and fulfilling.

The future of women's health is rich with opportunity, and peptides are at the forefront of that transformation. By taking the first step, educating yourself, and committing to this process, you've already embraced a proactive approach to your health.

Trust your efforts, stay curious, and know that every bit of care you show yourself today paves the way for a healthier, brighter tomorrow. You have the tools, knowledge, and power to shape your wellness journey—now, it's time to keep moving forward.

FAQs

What are peptides, and how do they work?

Peptides are short chains of amino acids that act as signaling molecules in the body, instructing cells to perform specific functions. For women, peptides can help with a range of goals, including hormonal balance, skin rejuvenation, improved sleep, fat loss, and enhanced energy. They work by mimicking or boosting the body's natural processes, such as stimulating growth hormone production or promoting collagen synthesis.

Are peptides safe to use?

When used responsibly and under the guidance of a healthcare provider, peptides are generally safe and well-tolerated. However, like any supplement or treatment, they come with potential side effects, such as mild nausea, headaches, or injection site irritation (if injectable). Consulting a professional ensures proper dosing and helps mitigate risks.

How long does it take to see results from peptides?

The timeline for visible results varies depending on the peptide and your specific goals. For instance, peptides for skin rejuvenation, like GHK-Cu, may show noticeable improvements in a few weeks. Growth hormone-releasing peptides, like CJC-1295, might take 8-12 weeks for measurable improvements in energy, body composition, or sleep quality. Consistency is key!

Why should peptides be cycled?

Cycling peptides prevents the body from becoming desensitized to their effects and minimizes risks of overstimulation. Typically, peptides are taken in cycles lasting 4-12 weeks, followed by a break of equal or longer length. This approach ensures their continued effectiveness and reduces the likelihood of side effects.

How do I monitor my progress while using peptides?

Monitoring involves tracking both objective and subjective changes. Objective measures include metrics like body composition, skin texture, or lab results (e.g., hormone levels). Subjective measures include improvements in mood, energy levels, sleep quality, or focus. Keeping a journal or using an app can help capture these details and identify trends over time.

Can I combine peptides with other treatments or supplements?

Yes, peptides often complement other wellness practices, such as balanced nutrition, regular exercise, and skincare routines. However, combining peptides with other treatments (like hormone therapy or skincare products) should be done under the supervision of a healthcare provider to avoid interactions or overloading the body.

How do I get started with peptides?

The first step is consulting with a healthcare provider who understands peptides and your health history. They can recommend the best peptides for your goals, outline a safe dosing schedule, and provide guidance on cycling. Researching and purchasing high-quality peptides from trusted sources is also essential to ensure safety and effectiveness.

References and Helpful Links

What are peptides? (n.d.). WebMD.
https://www.webmd.com/a-to-z-guides/what-are-peptides

Radiance Age Management. (2024, September 25). Peptide supplementation for Women - Radiance age Management.
https://radianceantiaging.com/services/anti-aging-for-women/solution-integrated-age-management-program-for-women/peptide-supplementation-for-women/

Hubmed. (2025, February 27). Epitalon peptide: Unlocking the secrets of longevity.
https://www.hubmeded.com/blog/epitalon-peptide-the-secrets-of-longevity#:~:text=It%20is%20thought%20that%20the,environmental%20damage%2C%20or%20normal%20aging.

Sciacca, M. F., Naletova, I., Giuffrida, M. L., & Attanasio, F. (2022). Semax, a synthetic regulatory peptide, affects Copper-Induced abeta aggregation and amyloid formation in artificial membrane models. ACS Chemical Neuroscience, 13(4), 486–496.
https://doi.org/10.1021/acschemneuro.1c00707

8 best peptides for anti aging. (n.d.).
https://www.lavishrn.com/blog/best-peptides-anti-aging

Ld, L. S. M. R. (2019, January 23). 5 Evidence-Based Ways Collagen may improve your hair. Healthline. https://www.healthline.com/nutrition/collagen-for-hair

Caffeine and peptides: a powerful duo for your hair | Tresan International. (n.d.). https://tresan.com. https://tresan.com/en/blog/caffeine-and-peptides-a-powerful-duo-for-your-hair?srsltid=AfmBOooToyl1f0JZ9kN6bkPws-VSbDDfjb1o47PkECNY7P0WNxYoOfWw

www.ingramcontent.com/pod-product-compliance
Lightning Source LLC
LaVergne TN
LVHW012033060526
838201LV00061B/4586